Joy

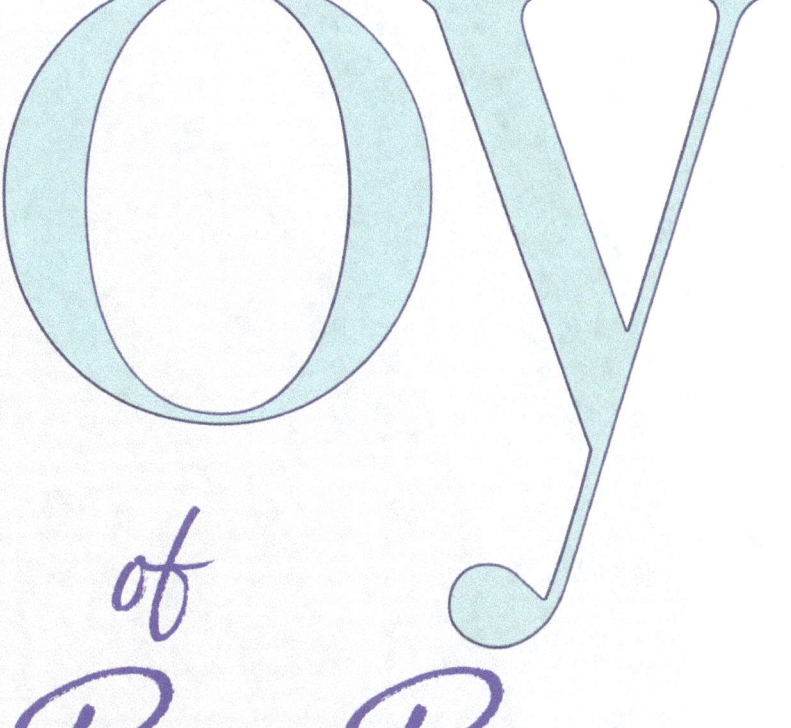

of
BonBons

Herbal Superfood Confections

Teresa Boardwine, RH (AHG)

Joy of BonBons

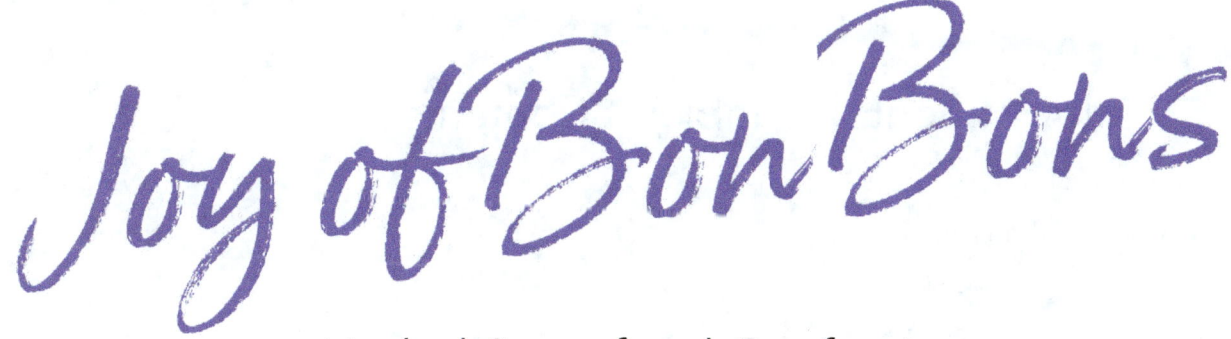

Herbal Superfood Confections

by

Teresa Boardwine, RH (AHG)

Green Comfort School of Herbal Medicine
www.greencomfortherbschool.com

Layouts by Tara Griffin

Joy of BonBons Table of Contents

BonBon Recipes from A-Z

Acknowledgments, Gratitude and Inspiration

The recipes that I am sharing with you are original creations, inspired by my lifetime love of real food, holistic healing and medicinal herbs. While teaching Home Economics in Germany I discovered herbs, natural gourmet cooking and holistic nutrition. My desire to incorporate the medicinal use of herbs led me to the California School of Herbal Studies. The journey returned me full circle to my Appalachian Mountain roots. Grandmother Ashworth, "Granny", inspired me with her gardens, apple orchard, concord grapes, flowers, chickens, homemade pies and creamed white corn. It was my mother who taught me the power of food and nutrition through my teenage years. When Kat Maier and I began our business, Dreamtime Center for Herbal Studies, I created the menus for each body system, developed apothecary labs and holistic nutrition classes. Reflecting now on my 30 years as an herbalist, and 40 years as a teacher, it has always been about food and healing. I have deep appreciation for the people and experiences that have influenced my teaching and inspired my journey.

I respectfully acknowledge that the sacred land I live upon is the traditional territory of the Shawandasse Tula, Shawanwaki, Shawnee and Manahoac Nations. Stewarding this land near Shenandoah National Park and the headwaters of the Rappahannock River is a great honor. It is my hope that the plants will continue to teach and heal us in this magical place. We have registered this beautiful space with the United Plant Savers as a Botanical Sanctuary for educational purposes.

My original inspiration to create BonBons is from Rosemary Gladstar. Her recipe for "Magic Zoom Balls" in her book, "The Science and Art of Herbalism", became an early favorite of mine. As Rosemary once said to me, "once you change an ingredient it is your own". She encouraged me to be playful with the original recipe and inspired me to have fun creating my own versions. You can make your own versions of my recipes as you make substitutions and experiment with a variety of powdered herbs. Thanks Rosemary for the inspiration and your sparkle!

At **Green Comfort School of Herbal Medicine,** I love teaching my students to make BonBons. I am grateful that students of the plants have sustained me over the years. And I am delighted to have had the opportunity to teach so many about using plants as foods and medicine. Making bonbons is a fun part of our gatherings for friends and community. I have created these superfood confections to build stamina, increase resilience, boost alertness and fortify wellness, but also to just have fun! My desire is to spark the "Joy of BonBons" within everyone. Thanks for sharing the journey with me.

I am fortunate to have found joy in teaching herbal medicine and connecting people to plants.

Gratefully yours,

Teresa

Joy of Bon Bons defined

Bon, "Good" or BonBon, meaning "Good good" is the literal French interpretation. The etymology of the word bon, is a wonderful place to begin. The feminine form of bon/good is bonne and bon is from the Latin bonus. Definitions mostly suggest a BonBon to be a small confection, often with a chocolate base. The center can be filled with liqueur, nuts or sweet ingredients, such as dates. It may also contain ganache, caramel, or nougat. The definition from Merriam-Webster.com is "something that is pleasing in a light or frivolous way".

It is with joy that I use this definition of BonBon to create these tasty confections in a "light and frivolous way". For me that is an invitation to play and to find new and exciting ways to create herbally infused confections. My goal for this book is to create recipes incorporating medicinal herbs to be ingested as food. My passion is the process of creating and formulating in this case, BonBons. My directive, from the goddess, is to inspire the creation of BonBons in herbal apothecaries and homes as a medicinal confection to build stamina, improve digestion, spark the fires of reproductive health and have a good time. The recipes inspired here are delicious morsels of goodness, packed with herbs and fueled by Joy!

I define the BonBon to be a superfood confection in rolled balls of goodness.

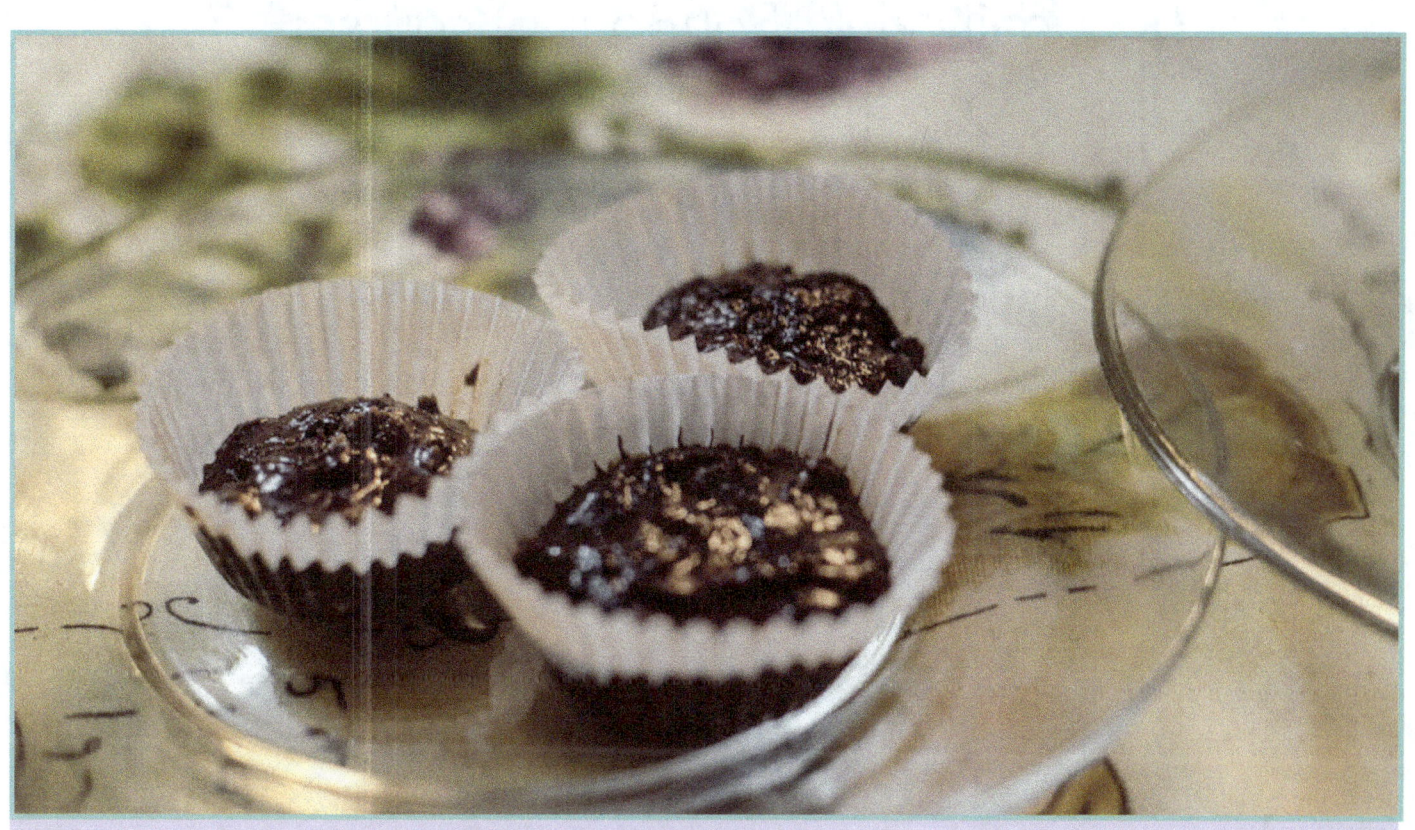

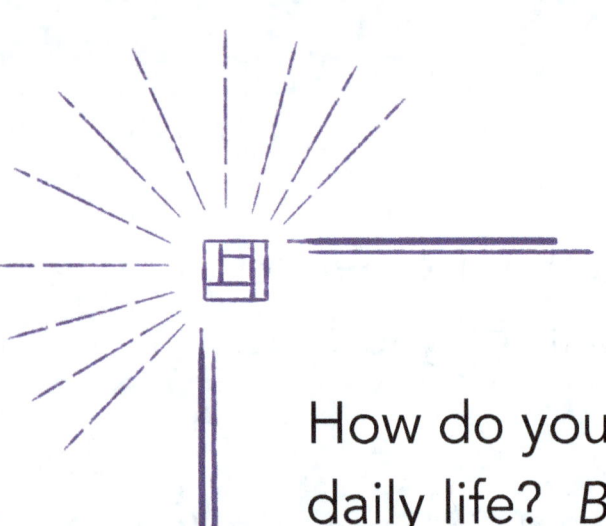

How do you add herbs into your daily life? *BonBons* of course!

Herbs used in our recipes are food and medicine. As an herbalist and consumer of botanical medicine, it is my goal to encourage others to mix and match the herbs to meet individual needs and desires. Consult the list of powdered herbs to help you decide based on a short description of health benefits and actions. If you are not familiar with the plants research using several sources to assure the right one for you. Create one or two recipes that contain adaptogens or brain fuel herbs and yummy ingredients.

As a practitioner of herbal medicine, I like to introduce this way to consume herbs as food to nourish, balance and support. These recipes are not meant to treat disease. All of the herbs chosen lend themselves to be ingested as part of the dietary intake with nut butters and good oils. All the BonBon recipes are gluten free, mostly paleo, all can be easily made vegan and require no baking.

What a treat! What a cool way to get a nutritional boost for a busy life. Keep a batch made and in the refrigerator for the grab and go life. To Go BonBons!

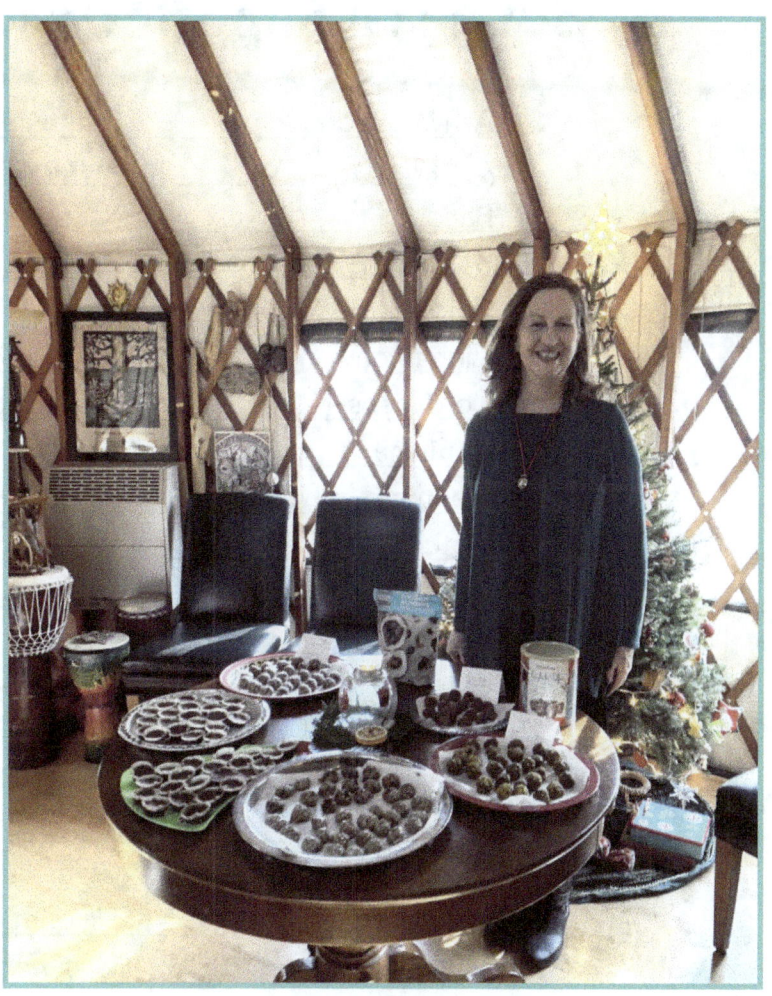

Botanical Superfood Powders:

Ashwagandha	*Withania somnifera*
Astragalus	*Astragalus membranaceous*
Bacopa	*Bacopa monnieri (Brahmi)*
Baobab	*Baobab Adansonia digitata*
Chlorella	*Chlorella vulgaris*
Cinnamon	*Cinnamomum verum, ceylon*
Cordyceps	*Cordyceps militaris*
Damiana	*Tunera diffusa*
Eleuthero	*Eleutherococcus senticosus*
Gotu Kola "Brahmi"	*Centella asiatica*
Guarana	*Paullnia cupana*
Holy Basil	*Ocimum sanctum*
Kola Nut	*Cola acuminate*
Licorice	*Glycyrrhiza glabra*
Lucuma	*Pouteria lucuma*
Maca	*Lepidium meyenii*
Matcha green tea	*Camellia sinensis*
Milk Thistle seed	*Silybum marianum*
Mucuna	*Mucuna pruriens*
Reishi	*Ganoderma lucidum*
Rose	*Rosa carina or gallica*
Shatavari	*Asparagus racemosus*
Solomon's seal	*Polygonatum multiflorum*
Turmeric	*Curcuma longa*

Cordyceps
sinensis
powder ~ organic
Astragalus
membranaceaus
powder
Eleuthero
senticosus
Ashwagandh
powder
Shatavari
powder
Maca

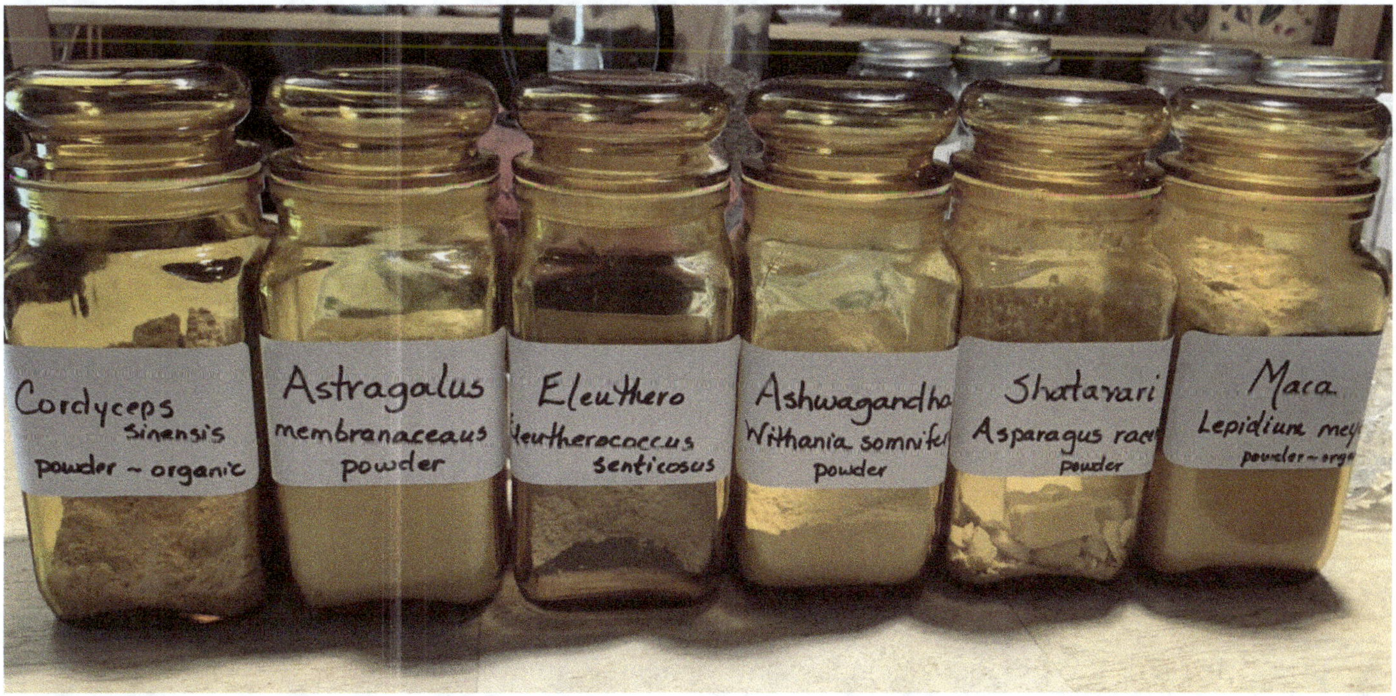

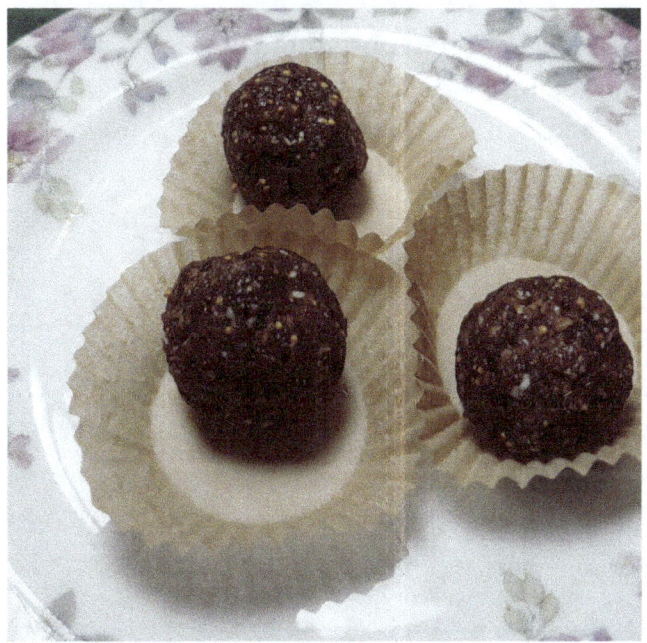

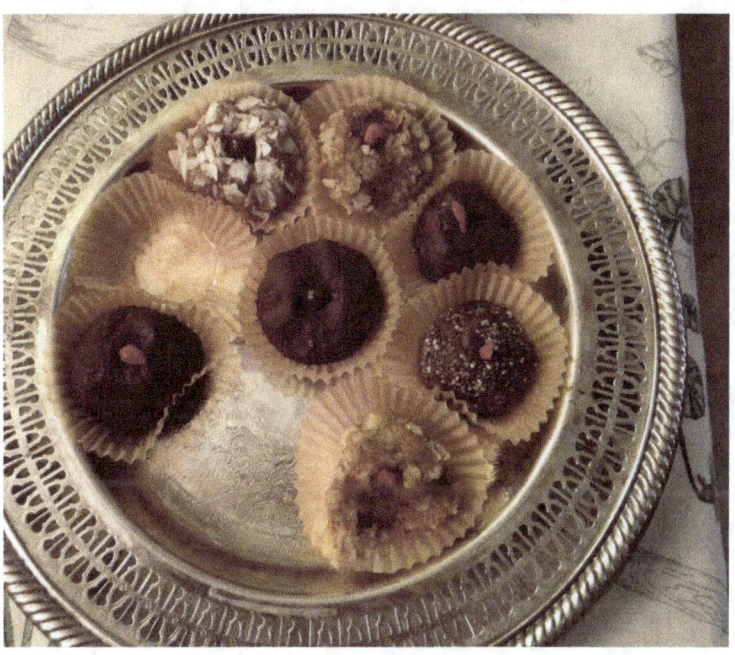

Botanical Superfood Attributes and Actions

A short description to help you determine which herbs as food might serve you best. Remember to read about them in several herb books and websites for more information.

Ashwagandha *Withania somnifera* This root is known as "Winter Cherry" for the summer fruit but it is the root we use, harvested in the fall. It is an adaptogen, raising vitality, balancing hormones, boosting immunity and promoting sleep.

Astragalus *Astragalus membranaceous* A nourishing tonic root that taste sweet and warm. It is known to stimulate phagocytes which clean up debris and helps to produce our innate anti-viral interferon.

Bacopa *Bacopa monnieri*, "Brahmi", known in India for nervous system disorders including epilepsy. As a memory stimulant it is said to increase acuity, repair neuronal pathways and reduce inflammation. The presence of steroidal saponins justifies the claims for arthritis, asthma and rheumatic conditions.

Baobab *Adansonia digitate* Fruit of the upside-down tree is edible, has a citrus flavor and is a good source of vitamin C, potassium, carbohydrates, and phosphorus. Baobab seed powder is used in foods because of its nutrients, health benefits, and as a natural preservative.

Chlorella *Chlorella vulgaris* is a species of green microalga used as a protein-rich food additive.

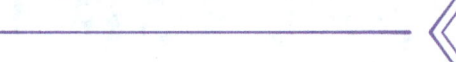

Cinnamon *Cinnamomum verum* is rich in volatile oils known to be anti-viral, antibacterial and anti-fungal. It is a warming and stimulating as food that affects cardio. The meta-analysis shows significant reduction in fasting blood glucose in insulin resistance. And it smells like Christmas and snickerdoodles.

Cordyceps *Cordyceps militaris, sinensis* As a combination of caterpillar and mushroom it has traditionally been used to enhance vigor and vitality. It is known to help with oxygen exchange in the alveoli. It can enhance the immune system, increase endurance and build stamina.

Damiana *Tunera diffusa* is the feel good herb, relaxes the nervous system while toning the reproductive organs, some say it is an aphrodisiac, enjoy the bonbon effect.

Eleuthero *Eleutherococcus senticosus* the herb that coined the term adaptogen. It is used to increase endurance, build stamina and nourish the adrenal glands. Builds resilience to stress.

Gotu Kola *Centella asiatica "Brahmi"* a longevity herb that is also a connective tissue tonic. Known as a brain tonic to help with focus and memory.

Guarana *Paullinia cupana* seed of the fruiting vine contains xanthines including caffeine, theobromine and theophylline, also tannins and saponins. For short term energy.

Holy Basil *Ocimum sanctum* herb is sacred to the goddess Lakshmi, protects the heart from stress and is taken as an adaptogen to boost immune resistance while promoting clarity of mind.

Kola Nut *Cola acuminate* seed is used to stimulate alertness encourages muscular strength, counters lethargy and used as an anti-depressant.

Maca *Lepidium meyenii* is known as Peruvian ginseng, it's an edible root in the Brassica family that is native in the high Andes mountains. Maca powder may be raw, or gelatinized to be used as a superfood in smoothies and bonbons.

Matcha green tea *Camellia sinensis* is the tea plant that offers strong antioxidant polyphenols useful as a protective stimulant that promotes longevity.

Milk Thistle seed *Silybum marianum* shown to protect the liver from harm of alcohol and poisons, this seed is useful to include in food as a liver rejuvenative.

Mucuna *Mucuna Pruriens* extract is a Dopamine Booster that is rich in antioxidants and may help support overall brain and cognitive function and help promote a healthy mood. It may also promote healthy sleep, aid libido, and contribute to sexual health.

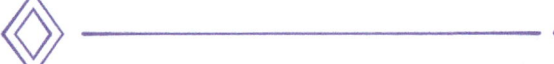

Reishi *Ganoderma lucidum* As a woody mushroom it needs to be processed to be digestible. It contains polysaccharides including beta glucan which boost the immune function and also is anti-inflammatory and liver protective. In TCM it is used to protect the Shen or Spirit Force.

Rose *Rosa gallica* is a remedy for depression and used in food as rosewater and organic petals to gladden the heart, it is astringent, use sparingly.

Shatavari *Asparagus racemosus* promotes fertility and acts a sexual tonic. Known as the herb of 100 spouses, it is a nutritive immune support.

Solomon's seal *Polygonatum multiflorum* the sweet tasting tuber is sued for the tendons to reduce inflammation in the joints and considered a yin tonic.

Turmeric *Curcuma longa root provides one of the best anti-inflmmatories as food and medicine. Research shows it lowers sticky platelets which lessens blood clots and helps reduce lactic acid accumulation.*

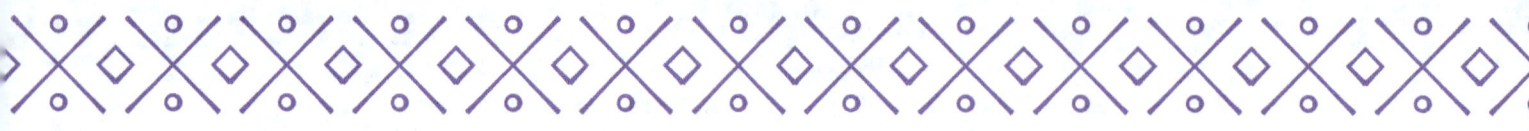

Dry Ingredients:

Nut butters:
Almond
Cashew
Hazelnut
Peanut butter
Pumpkin seed
Sunflower seed
Tahini
Walnut

Fats:
Almond paste
Cocoa butter
Coconut Cream
Coconut mana
Coconut oil
Ghee

Sweeteners:
Chocolate chips
Confectioner's sugar
Honey
Maple syrup
Maple syrup crystals
Rice syrup
Vegetable glycerin

Dried Fruit:
Apricots
Cherries
Coconut
Cranberries
Crystalized Ginger
Date
Figs
Goji berries

Nuts and Seeds:
Almonds
Cashews
Chia seeds
Hemp seeds
Pecans
Pumpkin seeds
Walnuts
Sesame seeds
Sunflower seeds

Liquid Ingredients:
Amaretto Liqueur
Almond extract
Cherry Liqueur
Honey
Maple extract
Maple Syrup
Rice Syrup
Vanilla extract

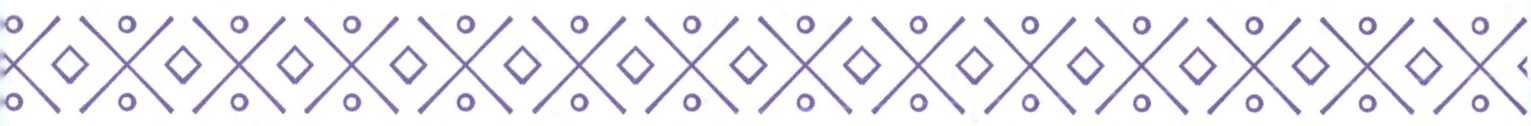

BonBon Ingredient List

Apple Pie Spice
Black pepper
Cacao powder
Cardamom powder
Cayenne powder
Chia seeds
Chocolate Chips
Cinnamon powder
Cocoa butter
Cocoa Crisps
Cacao nibs
Cacao powder
Coconut flakes
Coconut mana
Coconut milk powder
Coconut oil
Espresso
Ginger powder
Hemp protein
Hemp seeds
Himalayan pink salt
Oats
Protein shake powder
Pumpkin Pie Spice
Vanilla powder (optional)
Whey

Measurement /Abbreviations

T	Tablespoon
t	teaspoon
c	Cup
pwd	powder
oz.	ounce
ml	milliliters

Equipment:

Double Boiler
Sauce pan
Mixing bowls
Soup bowls
Spoons
Rubber spatula
Dry measuring cup set
Liquid measuring cup (1 – 2c)
Measuring spoons
Whisk
Food processor

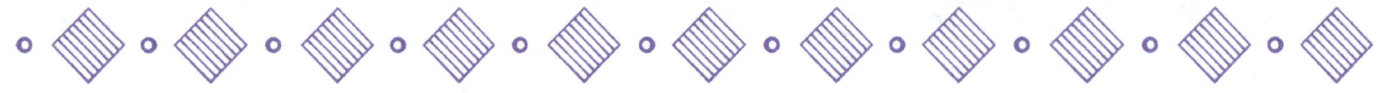

Forming the BonBons

- Mix the ingredients in a bowl or double boiler.
- To harden the bonbon mix, place in the refrigerator or freezer for a few minutes.
- When processing denser ingredients, nuts, dates, dried fruits and crystalized ginger, use a food processor
- Use disposable food grade gloves.
- To form into balls without sticking, drop a bit of oil onto gloved hands and rub together.
- Teresa often uses the two spoon technique during demonstrations or in class for a quick medicinal treat forming irregular balls of yumminess
- Scoop out to roll with different size of scoops; small melon baller, large melon baller, ice cream scoop and or a meat ball scoop.
- Choose the size of the ball in correspondence to the amount of recipe made and the desired consumption. Some of the recipes are meant to be only 1 bite, so make them small enough to go into the mouth comfortably.
- For large Bonbons use stiffer ingredients, like dates, nuts and fillers to form ones that you can bite into.

Enjoy making bonbons.

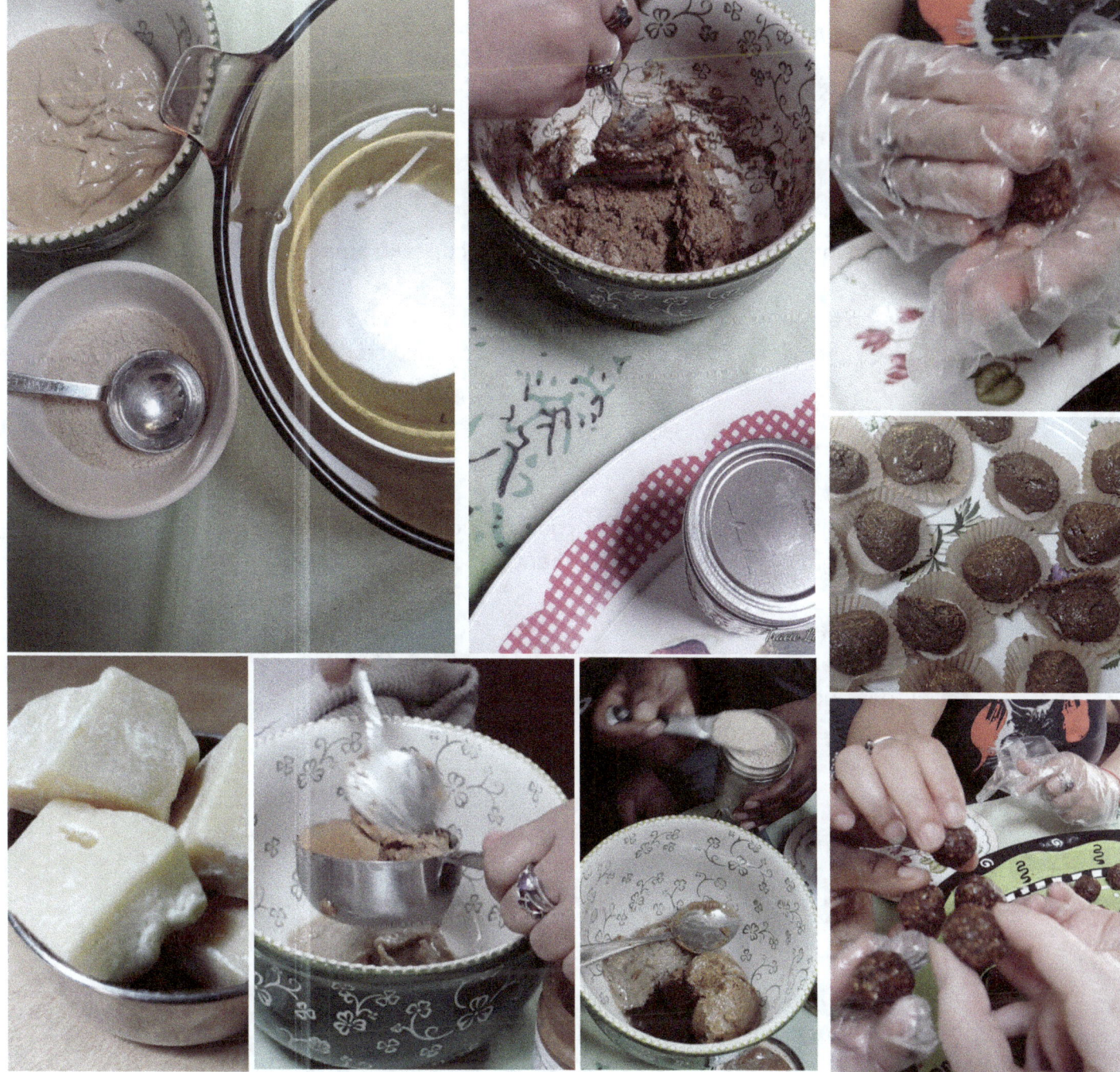

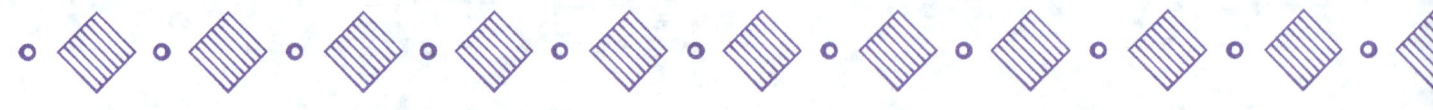

Serving

Place them into candy cups, mini unbleached cupcake cups or just into a candy box.
Arrange on a platter, use paper doily for a pop of color or seasonal interest.
May be arranged by recipe on a tired tea or cupcake stand.

Storing

Store in Air-Tight container for later consumption.
Line an air-tight container with parchment paper or waxed paper at the bottom
and in between layers.
Include a paper towel in the container to absorb moisture.
Label to include the ingredients and date made.
Store in the refrigerator in an air-tight container for up to 2 weeks.

Freeze for up to 1 month.
Place in the refrigerator for 15-30 minutes to thaw out before serving.

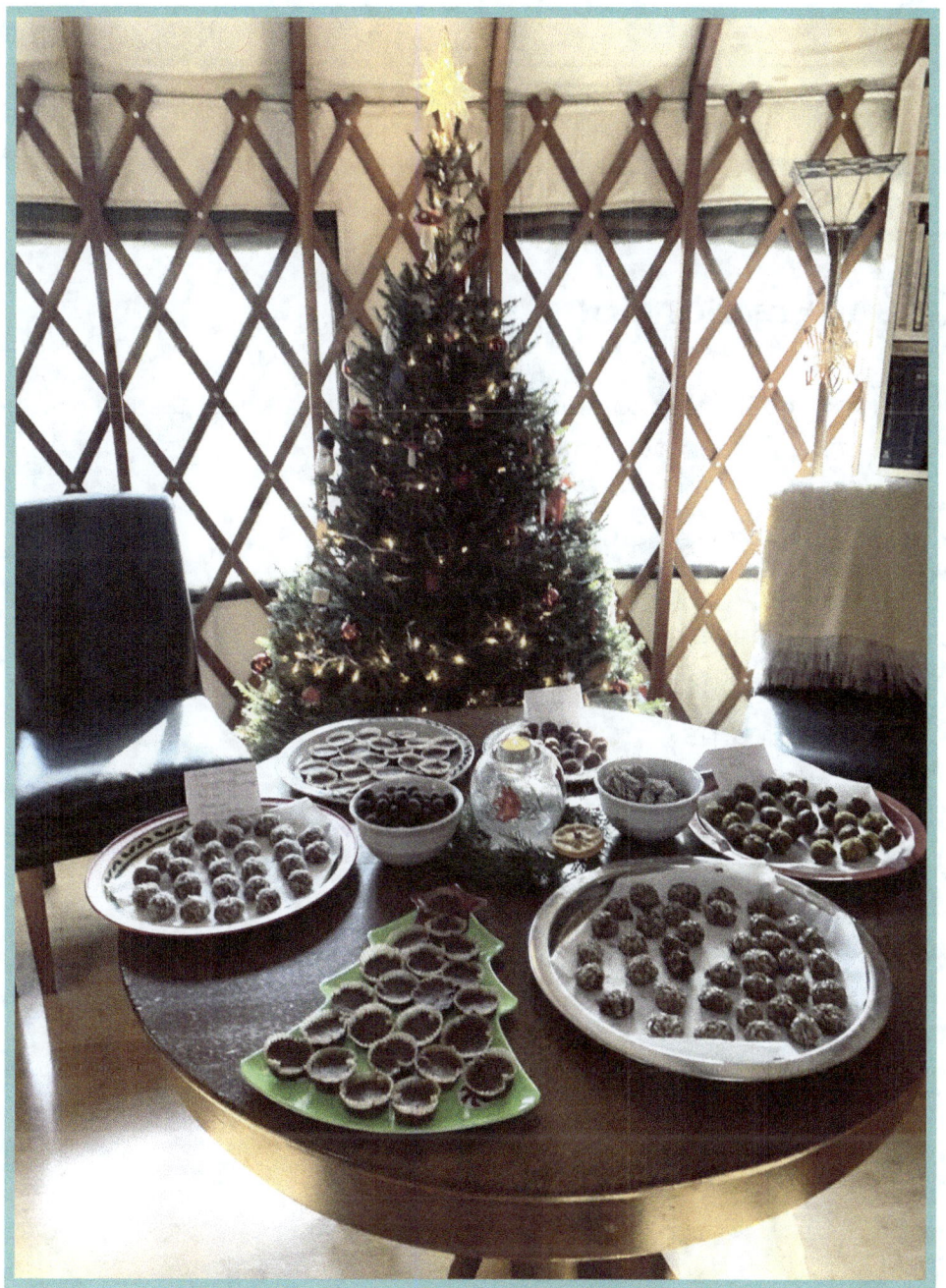

Almandine BonBon

This delicious confection combines the almond with sweet tasting root herbs to boost immunity and build stamina.

1 c	Blanched almonds soaked
8 oz	Almond Paste, one box or 12 T.
1 T	Amaretto Liqueur or
1 t	Almond extract
2 T	Lucuma
2 T	Astragalus
1 c	Slivered Almonds to cover
1 c	Coconut, unsweetened to cover

Directions:

Soak the blanched almonds in water for several hours in the refrigerator.
Rinse and drain completely. Dry nuts on a tea towel.
Grind Almonds in a food processor.
Add Almond paste, almond extract or amaretto and continue processing to combine all the ingredients well.
Add the powdered herbs; Astragalus and Lucuma At this point if the mixture is runny or too dry it will be hard to shape into balls.
Either add more liquid almond flavor if too dry or add a bit more herb powders if it is too wet.
To firm, Place in the refrigerator or freezer for a few minutes.
Shape the mixture into small balls, one bite size.
Roll some in each; slivered almonds or coconut flakes
Arrange on a platter or store in container for later consumption.

May be served with a bit of Amaretto or hot chai tea.

Almond Joy–ish BonBon

One of my guilty pleasures enjoyed on occasion has been the Almond Joy. The taste of the coconut and the almond on top does insight joy in me. I am introducing my version as a delightful substitute with the added benefit of medicinal mushrooms, Lion's Mane and Reishi.

¾ c	Coconut manna
½ c	Honey
1 t	Vanilla
1 c	Shredded Coconut
2 T	Lion's Mane
2 T	Reishi Powder
¼ c	Cacao butter
½ c	Cocoa Powder
2 T	Maple syrup
	Dash of salt
	Almonds for the top of each

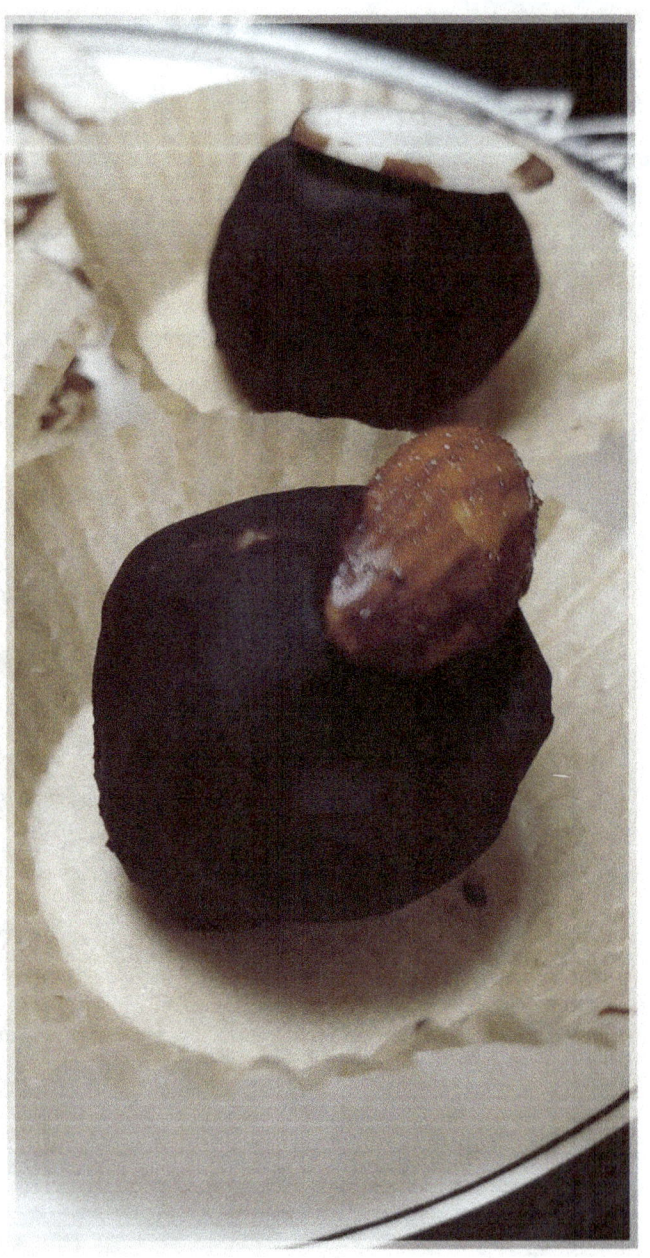

Directions:

On low heat, melt: coconut manna, and honey

Remove from heat, and whisk in Honey, Vanilla and Salt

Mix in the Lion's Mane & Reishi.

Add shredded coconut.

Refrigerate.

In a second saucepan, melt cocoa butter, add the cocoa powder and maple syrup. add more of either to get the right consistency.

Roll the coconut centers into balls using gloved hands.

Drop each into the cooled cocoa to coat, then

Place each dipped bonbon onto a wire rack to cool.

Place the almond on top.

Set in fridge to harden.

When set take out and put into storage container. Store in the refrigerator.

Enjoy the Almond Joy-ish guilty pleasure moments. Ahhh!

Brahmi Cacao Bites

Brahmi derives from Sanskrit and translates as "energy of universal consciousness." Gotu Kola in the north of India and Bacopa in the south of India are called Brahmi. Gotu Kola and Bacopa affect the mind and consciousness.

4 T	Coconut oil
¼ c	Cacao butter
½ t	Cinnamon pwd
½ t	Cardamom
pinch	Himalayan pink salt
½ c	Maple syrup
1 t	Vanilla extract
4 T	Cacao, raw pwd
2 T	Gotu Kola Brahmi
2 T	Bacopa Brahmi
½ c	Walnuts, crushed

Directions:

In a sauce pan, melt the coconut oil and cacao butter.

Add the cinnamon, cardamom, spices and salt. Allow them to warm until you smell them.

Turn off the heat.

Add vanilla and maple syrup. Blend with whisk.

Mix together Cacao and Brahmi. Add a Tablespoon at a time, until it is the right consistency.

Add the Walnuts into the batter. It should stiffen easily with the nuts, if not, refrigerate for 30 minutes.

Roll into bite size balls. Lightly sprinkle with pink salt.

Enjoy with a cup of Holy Basil "Tulsi" tea with a sprinkle of Roses. A great meditative way to align your mind, body and spirit for your day.

Brain Boosting BonBon

For focused attention, greater recall and memory enhancement, consider this intriguing herbal confection. Green tea is a polyphenol rich super food and both Lion's Mane and Bacopa help with neuronal repair and cognition. Plus, it tastes good!

In a food processor, mix these ingredients until a paste forms.

1 c	Walnut butter
½ c	Walnuts, processed into small pieces
½ t	Vanilla bean powder or extract
3 T	Maple crystals
1T	MCT Oil, stream in

Measure out and blend the powders together:

1 T	Matcha Green Tea powder
2 T	Lion's Mane powder
1 T	Bacopa powder

Add a Tablespoon of the herbal blend into the paste at a time until the mixture is well blended. Roll into balls and lay them out on parchment paper. For Toppings to roll… Lightly sift Match with maple crystals over them
   ½ c   Walnuts, ground
   ½   2 T Matcha & 1 T maple crystal
Refrigerate to set. Enjoy 1 or 2 bonbons a day for super alert energy boost.

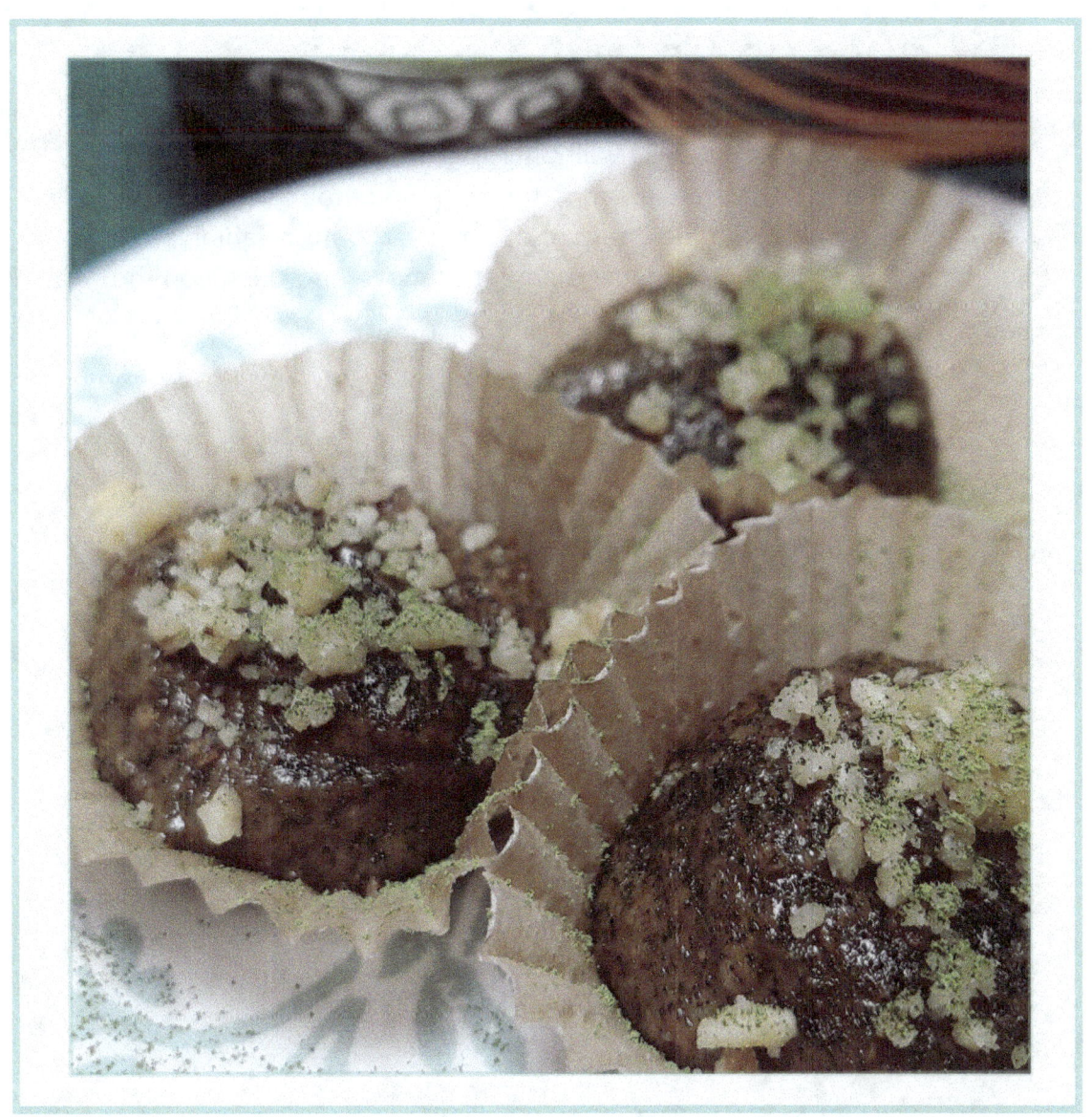

Chai & Yoga BonBon

This delicious confection rolls traditional yogi tea herbs and spices into a superfood delight. Reduce inflammation with Solomon's seal and Turmeric as we build stamina with Eleuthero. Sesame seed butter, Tahini, and sesame seeds ground and balance the air element to move effortlessly on the yoga mat.

3 T	Solomon's seal pwd
2 T	Eleuthero pwd
1 T	Turmeric pwd
1 t	Ginger pwd
¼ t	Black pepper, ground
1 T	Coconut milk pwd.
1 c	Coconut manna
2 T	Rice Syrup
½ c	Tahini
¼ c	Chia seeds *also known as Salvia hispanica*
½ c	Sesame seeds, toasted

Directions:

Mix powders together and set aside.

Warm the Cocoa mana in a double boiler.

Add Rice syrup and Tahini to warmed mixture and blend well.

To hydrate the Chia seeds add them into the warm mixture.

Then add the Powdered herbs a little at a time while blending.

To reach the desired consistency add a thin stream of warm water.

In the water one could add a flavoring agent, like maple extract or almond extract.

Add just enough moisture to be able to blend in the powders.

Set in the refrigerator to chill.

Chai w/ Yoga BonBon continued...

In a dry skillet toast the sesame seeds, when they begin to pop keep them moving until you smell toasted sesame.

When the mixture is ready to roll into bonbons scoop out a rounded teaspoonful and roll it in your gloved hand until soft again and then roll in the toasted sesame seeds.

Press the sesame seeds into the bonbon.

Arrange them in unbleached muffin cups and box.

Enjoy with a cup of Chai Latte before yoga class.

Namaste

Cherry Almond Truffles

Make these little morsels for when you need a cherry on top.

1 c   Cherries, dried
2 c   Almonds, whole not roasted or salted
1 c   Dates, pitted and chopped
4 T   *Ashwagandha* "Winter Cherry" powder
1 T   Almond flavoring or Cherry Liqueur

In a food processor process the almonds until finely ground. Add in the dates and dehydrated cherries. Process again until the mixture begins to clump together.

Add powdered herb, process. Add a bit of almond extract or cherry flavored liqueur to blend to perfect consistency. Using a tablespoon, scoop out even sized balls, and roll between greased hands to shape.
Store in the refrigerator for up to 3 days. Produces two dozen bonbons.
Serve with fresh cherries, dried cherries or canned black cherries
May be enjoyed with Cherry liqueur or a bowl full of cherries.

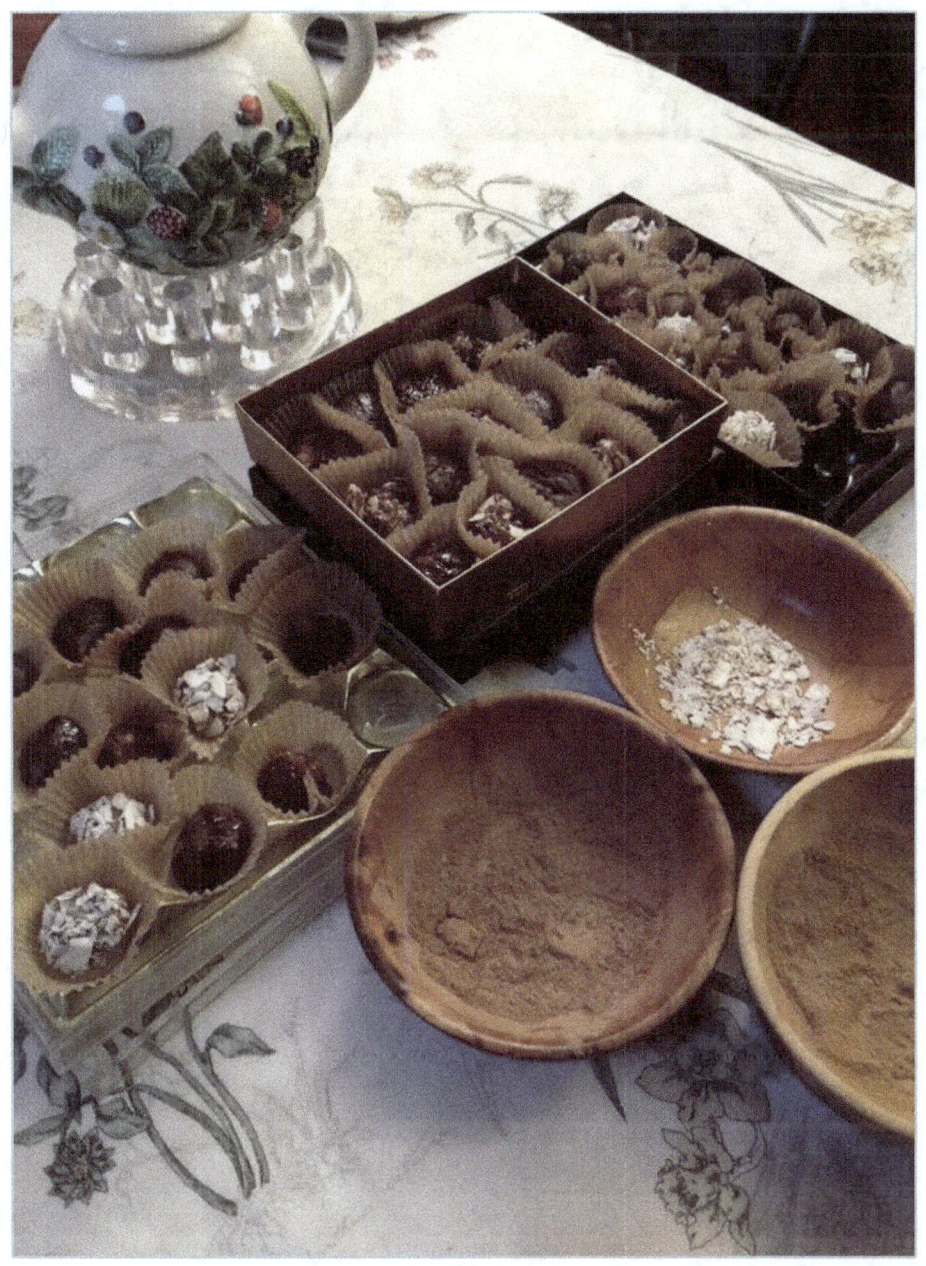

Chocolate Chili BonBon

The ancient Mayan civilization loved their spicy chocolate brew consisting of water, cacao beans, vanilla, honey, and chili peppers. They believed that it possessed spiritual qualities and worshiped their cacao god. These bonbons are a spicy stimulating reminder of how our journey with Cacao began.

¾ c	Cocoa Butter
¼ c	Coconut oil
½ c	Honey
1 t	Vanilla extract
1 c	Raw cacao powder
1 T	Cayenne
1 t	Chili powder (less if you can't take the heat.)
Pinch	Himalayan pink salt (Optional)

Directions:

Melt cocoa butter and coconut oil in a double boiler. When melted, turn off the heat.   Add honey and vanilla, whisk to mix.
Add Cacao powder, with Cayenne powder, may hold back some to dust the bonbon if you roll them.   (Optional Pinch of Salt)

Roll into bite size portions, dust with extra powder before serving.   Or choose a silicon mold that is bite size one. I have a flower mold and a star mold, you decide.
Pour into molds using a stainless spoon while slightly warm and still flowing and refrigerate to harden, make take an hour.

To serve turn out onto a smooth surface serving platter.
May want to accentuate the heat with a hot pepper flake on top of each.

This Bonbon is a great for invigorating warmth and stimulating blood flow before a work out, on a cold day and just for the heat of it!
Best served with water, But could pair with red wine.

Cinnamon, Spice & Everything Nice Bonbon

This delicious herbal delight is reminiscent of fall festivals. The apple pie spice flavors hide the fact it is also full of sugar balancing cinnamon and anti-inflammatory Turmeric and Yucca. This bonbon is sure to be a favorite for active folks who monitor sugar and avoid chocolate.

1 c	Pecans
1 c	Dates, pitted
½ c	Oats
1 t	Cinnamon
1 t	Turmeric
1 T	Lucuma
1 T	Yucca
2 t	Apple pie spice
1 t	water, enough moisture to bind the bonbon

Coating :
1 T	Cinnamon
1 T	Maple sugar crystals

Directions:

In a food processor, grind the nuts until small crumbs form.

Add the dates, process.

Mix all the powders together and spoon into the processor as it is running.

Drizzle a little warm water as needed to bind.

Add 1-2 teaspoons water to make dough stick to your hands.

Shape into quarter-size balls.

To coat, mix the cinnamon and sugar in a bowl,

Roll the balls in the mix to coat all over.

Store for 1 – 2 /day consumption.

May serve with Rooibos Chai tea for added warmth and aroma.

Enjoy!

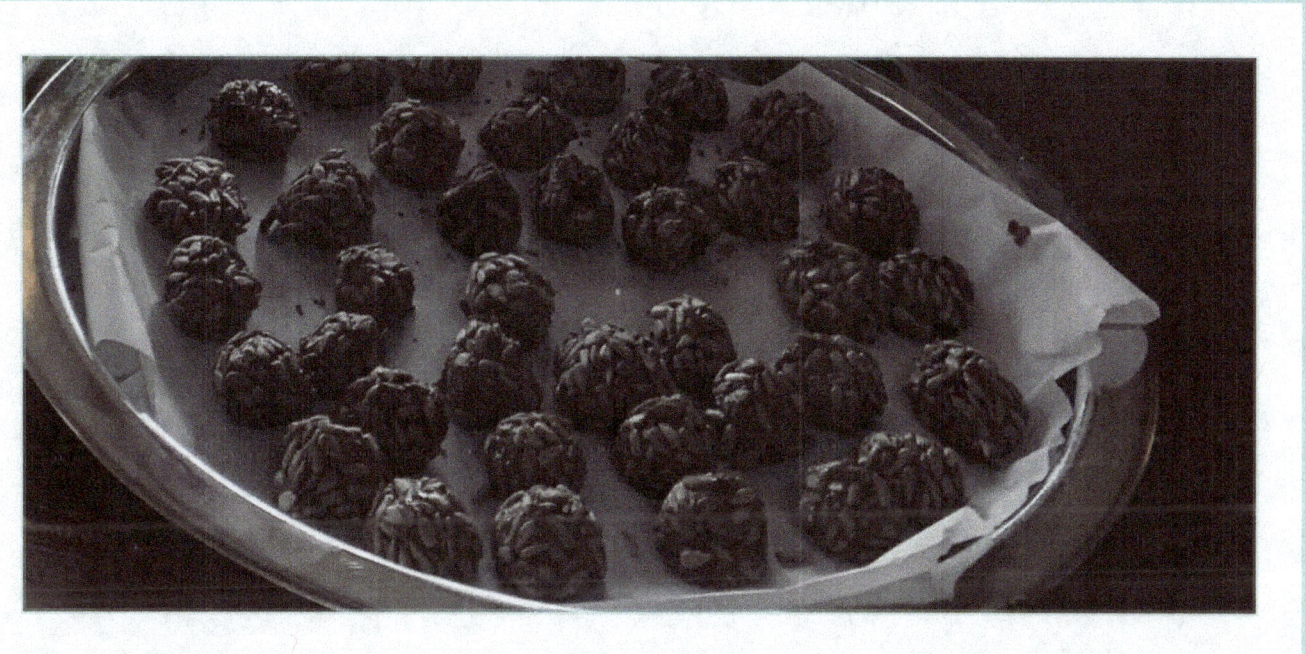

Cacao "Sang" Truffles

Super energizing chocolate bonbon, as close to a truffle as my expertise allows combines of my favorite plants American Ginseng (Sang) an extremely yin fortifying adaptogen and Cacao (Chocolate) a super food which offers heart opening stimulants. It is sure to be exciting!

½ c	Cashew butter
¼ c	Cacao butter
¼ c	Honey
½ t	Vanilla extract
⅓ c	Coconut flour
2 T	American ginseng powder
½ c	Chocolate Chunks
	or ganache (see recipe below)
	Cacao powder to dust

Melt the coconut and cacao butter over double boiler.

Add in the Ginseng powder mixing well.

Then add the Cashew nut butter, honey and vanilla until the mixture is thick. Refrigerate to allow the mixture to solidify.

Make the ganache recipe below:

Ganache

Ganache is the dense chocolate interior of the truffle made of chocolate and cream. I use the following recipe to form the dark chocolate ball of ganache.

| ½ c | Coconut milk |
| 1 c | Chocolate 72% |

Warm the coconut milk to blend in the cream. Then measure out the ½ c.

Next add the cup of chocolate discs to the milk and put the lid on the saucepan.
After 30 min. begin to stir in the middle to emulsify by starting in the center until the color changes and it becomes glossy.

Then stir in a wider circle to allow the chocolate to be blended together and melted to creamy texture.

Let it set for as long as it takes to cool and stiffen. It needs to cool gently for the ganache to form into the dense delicious center.

Form uniform small melon ball size ganache with gloved hands.

Remove the ginseng/coconut bonbon mixture from the refrigerator.
Using gloved hands form a bit of it around the smaller ball of ganache.
Dust with Cocoa powder through a sieve or roll them in a bowl of cocoa.
Place on parchment paper. Store the super sang truffles in an airtight container. Enjoy one or two a day a boost!

Keenan Sherwood @eatingwealthy was kind enough to teach me how to make ganache. He uses coconut milk as to please the non-dairy palate. It is so delicious and easy to make, Although it cannot be rushed. It is all in the whisking and temperature controls for chocolatiers. Try his truffles for a true delight.

Fruit & Nut "Zoom" BonBons

Energy and stamina promoting while providing nutrition and fuel for your hike, bike ride or kayak trip.

1 c	Almonds
1 c	Figs
1 c	Dates, pitted)
1 T	Ginger, crystallized
1 t	Vanilla extract
2 T	Guarana pwd.
1 T	Kola pwd.
1 T	Maca pwd.
1 t	Cinnamon pwd.
½ t	Nutmeg pwd. (optional)
¼ t	Clove pwd. (optional)

Process each of the first 4 ingredients in the food processor.

Mix all the powdered ingredients together.

Add the Powdered herbs, blend.

Using the food service disposable gloves, with a bit of oil on them;

Roll into bite size portions

Lay on parchment paper or wax paper in a storage box or container.

Will store well for a few weeks.

Great for outdoor adventures, make these to Go!

Going a "Nuttin" BonBons

This hazelnut chocolate delicacy is rich and decadent.
It is an intentionally sourced blend of pure ingredients, with the added excitement of endocrine balancing herbs.

½ c	Hazelnut butter
½ c	Chocolate Hazelnut butter
¼ c	Cacao Butter
2 T	Honey
2 T	Shatavari
2 T	Ashwagandha
½ c	Mini Chocolate chips
	Hazelnuts or filberts (one per each bonbon)

Melt cacao butter in a saucepan on low heat.

Stir in both hazelnut butters.

Add honey to sweeten and add moisture.

Mix in the herb powders.

Add some chocolate chips.

Roll the balls with gloved hands and top with a nut.

This hazelnut chocolate delicacy is rich and decadent. Like the fertility celebrations of our ancestors, it is time to "Go a Nuttin".

Enjoy this as your newest ritual.

Indonesian Influenced Satay *BonBon*

I took Indonesian cooking classes in The Hague. This bonbon is influenced by Satay, spicy peanut sauce. This bonbon version integrates the exotic Indonesian spices into food as medicine. It has a nice texture and aroma with a kick of spice.

¼ c	Peanut butter
½ c	Tahini
1 t	Toasted Sesame seed oil
1 T	Maple syrup
1 T	Braggs amino acid,	add more if the blend is too dry at the end.
1 t	Garlic pwd
½ t	Szechwan pepper
¼ t	Cayenne pwd
¼ t	Cumin pwd
¼ t	Coriander pwd
1 T	Cordyceps
1 T	Reishi
	Sesame seeds, toasted to cover

In the food processor mix the nut butters. The Tahini makes it a dryer blend. Add the liquid ingredients and blend. Mix together the powdered spices and herbs, adding in little at a time until blended and stiff.

Scoop out a small melon ball size and roll in sesame seeds.

This spicy bonbon can be eaten as a snack or appetizer.

I think it pairs well with a shrub; A vinegar based beverage to aid digestion of the good fats. "Smakelijk Eten"

Kava Coconut Contentment *BonBons*

There is nothing like a fresh coconut! This is in honor of that fruit from the topics. Kava needs the coconut fat for the kavalactones to be active and extracted. The adaptogen, Eleuthero, feeds exhausted adrenals and builds resistance to stress. To feel calm and relaxed like you are on vacation try this delectable bite of contentment and exhale!

½ c	Coconut manna
¼ c	Coconut sugar
1 T	Kava pwd
1 T	Eleuthero pwd
1 t	Vanilla bean pwd or vanilla extract
1 c	Shredded Coconut

In a sauce pan melt the coconut manna.

Add the coconut sugar and mix to dissolve.

Add the Vanilla bean to the mixture.

Blend in the powdered herbs

Add coconut flakes to the mixture to stiffen.

Chill to congeal.

Roll into one-bite size bonbons.

You could also shape it into golf balls, ping pong balls, a baseball or a big softball for a celebratory event. In any case I think these will be a vacation favorite. Remember happy is for birthdays and contentment is the goal. Enjoy!

Lakshmi Goddess BonBons

Lakshmi is the Hindu goddess of wealth, good fortune, power, luxury, beauty, and fertility. She holds the promise of material fulfilment and contentment. And since she represents fertility, in what better recipe to include the herb "for a woman with 100 husbands"; My favorite, Shatavari!

1 c	Cashew butter
2 T	Ghee
2 T	Honey
2 t	Licorice pwd
2 t	Turmeric pwd
1 t	Cardamom pwd
2 T	Shatavari pwd
1 T	Holy Basil pwd

Mix the cashew butter with the ghee in a double boiler. Remove from heat and add honey. Add in all the dry ingredients and continue to blend until smooth. Roll into balls.

Adorn them with sprinkled herbs fit for a goddess. It is your choice.

Perhaps some cinnamon and maple crystals.

Rose petals and rose glycerite would be great accompaniments as well.

Place on a silver platter and take to the temple, women's group, picnic, or whatever the occasion.

May Gratitude & Blessings flow!

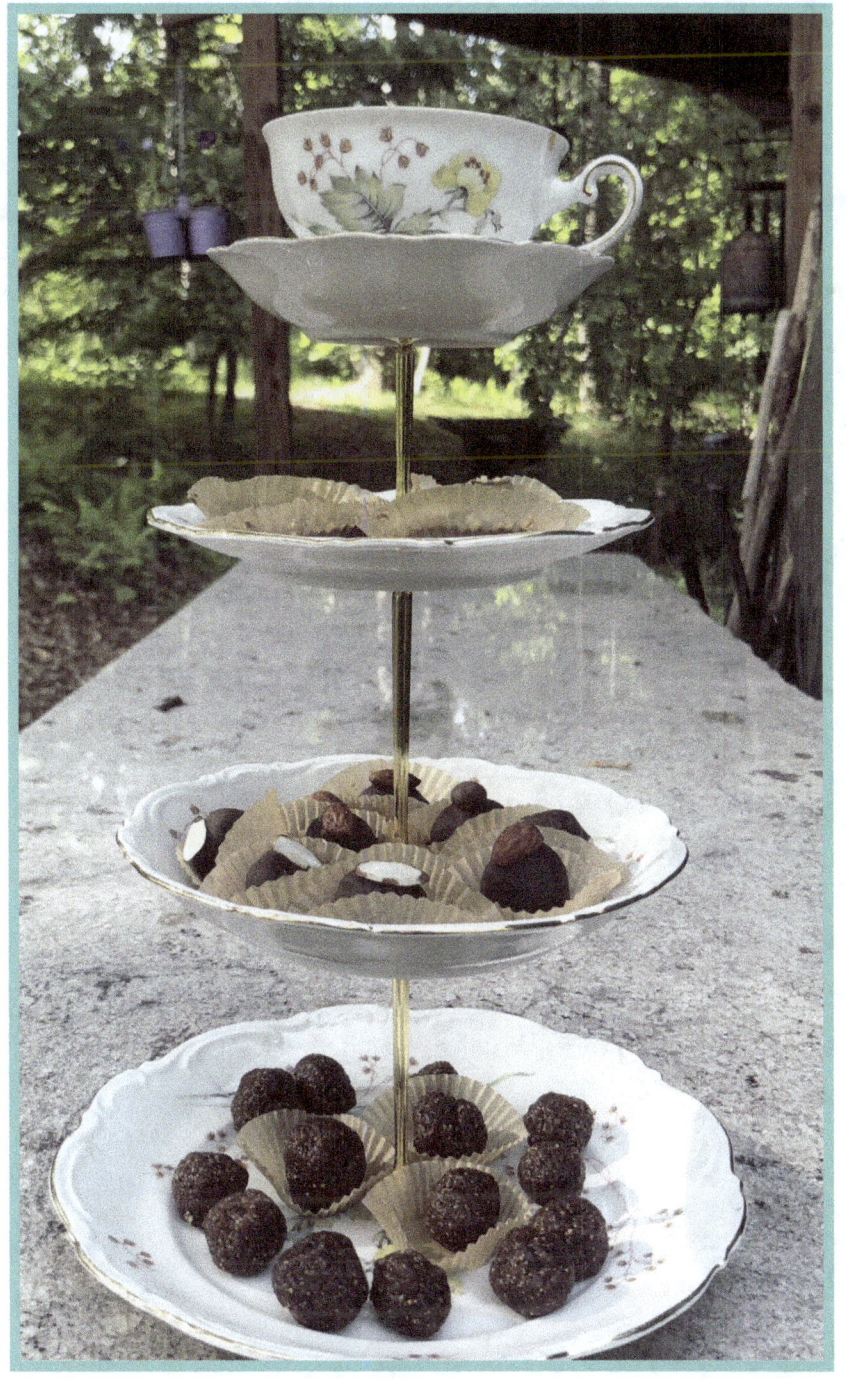

Maca Juana BonBon

This recipe uses sustainably harvested Sunflower seed butter which is super nutritious. Hemp, another super food plant from the *Cannabis* genus is rich in terpenes and cannabinoids for added health benefits. This bonbon can be made green by adding chlorella or nettles to boost chlorophyll.
Created for sheer pleasure, fortified by mother nature.

1 c   Sunflower seed butter
¼ c   Hemp Honey
¼ c   Hemp Collagen protein powder
2 T   Maca pwd
1 T   Mucuna pwd
1 T   Chlorella or Nettle pwd.
        Roll in roasted Hemp seeds & Sunflower seeds

Mix the sunflower seed butter together with the honey to form the base. Add the powders and mix together until the dough is stiff.
Using your food grade gloves, Rolling, Rolling, Rolling all the bonbons.
Best paired with music from the 70's.

Nutty Lemon Balls

I love lemon; the tartness, pucker power creating, clean smelling, happy making aroma and taste. This recipe will combine well with lemon ginger tea like a cookie or it can be used as a reward for getting your work done. Lemon is fresh!

1 c	Raw Almonds
1 c	Shredded Coconut
1 c	Almond Flour
3 T	Fresh Lemon Juice
2 T	Lemon Zest
2 T	Lemon Balm pwd
½ c	Honey
1 c	Coconut Cream, slighted warmed

Roast raw almonds in the oven at 350 for 10-12 minutes until fragrant. Cool on baking rack. Then add almonds to a food processor and process with almond flour and coconut until finely ground. Mix all other ingredients in a large measuring cup. Stream pour liquid ingredients into the processors while blending into dry ingredients. Put the entire mixture into the refrigerator or freezer for 10-15 minutes until the mixture is firm but pliable. bRoll into bite size balls with your gloved hands. Sprinkle a little extra lemon zest over each one. Enjoy the tartness with the nuts! It is a Fresh combination.

Pecan Date BonBons

These rich bonbons are a super nutritious food for everyday activity.

1 c	Dates, pitted
1 c	Pecans
½ c	Coconut, shredded flakes
6	Figs
4-6	Turkish Apricots
3 T	Ashwagandha
2 T	Maca
½ t	maple extract
1 T	Maple syrup

Process pecans in food processor until ground.

Add dates and other dried fruits including coconut.

process until mixture is sticky.

Add in the dry herbs and process.

Stream in the maple syrup and extract to add moisture, but not too much.

Roll into rather large balls and refrigerate until firm.

If they are sticky consider dusting them in:

Pecans, Oat flour, Cocoa or coconut flakes

Place them in cupcake papers to divide them in the refrigerator container.

Enjoy with hot tea or a refreshing ginger ale.

Renewable Energy BonBons

Let's build our own renewable energy grid. Build stamina, increase resistance to stress and improve your memory with this superfood recipe. Renewable energy is longer lasting.

2 T	Eleuthero
2 T	Astragalus
2 T	Cordyceps
2 T	Lion's Mane
1 c	Sunflower seed butter
¼ c	Ghee
¼ c	Rice Syrup
½ t	Himalayan pink salt
2 T	Chia seeds
1 T	Flax seeds
1 T	Sunflower seeds

First gather the powdered herbs and mix together 2 T each and store in a jar.
Warm the Ghee in a saucepan to liquify adding sunflower butter, salt and rice syrup.
Add 3 -4 Tablespoons of the renewable energy herbs and mix well.
Add the nuts and seeds to give bulk, add texture and provide energy.

Savory Power Balls

Power Ball sounds like a lottery winner. You can win better health through immuno-modulating Mushrooms in these easy to make savory snacks. Think salty, not sweet.

1 c	Tahini (sesame nut butter)
1 T	Miso
1 T	Nutritional Yeast
2 T	Reishi
2 T	Cordyceps
2 t	Bee Pollen
2 t	Dulce or Nori flakes
4 T	Sesame seeds, toasted

Mix in a bowl or food processor; Tahini, miso, nut yeast, mushroom powders.
If the mixture is too dry add a tablespoon of water or broth at a time to blend well.
Mix together the dry ingredients; Bee pollen, seaweed and sesame seeds.
Form processed ingredients into balls.
Roll balls to coat in dry ingredients.
Drop onto parchment paper for storing or onto a serving dish.

Eat 2-3 daily as a snack. Be sure to drink lots of water or hot tea as the tahini is hydrophilic and it demands a good amount of water to process. Try a good digestive tea of fennel, ginger and licorice. Enjoy!

Schweddy Rum Balls

Based on the 1998 SNL skit where two female co-anchors of NPR's "Delicious Dish" discuss Mr. Schweddy's holiday balls from his bakery, Season's Eatings. He asked the interviewers if they would like to try his Schweddy balls. All I can say here is, watch the skit to get the humor and hang on because we are re-creating the rum balls. Toast to frivolity!

8 oz	Vanilla Wafer Cookies
4 oz	Pecans, toasted
2 T	Ashwagandha or favorite adaptogen
½ c	Dark rum
3 T	Honey
¼ c	Cocoa powder
½ c	Confectioner's sugar

Process the vanilla wafer cookies in the food processor, add pecans.

Add adaptogen powder, rum and honey until well blended.

Add more nuts or rum as desired.

Grease hands as you want plenty of Lube.

Roll into meatball size balls.

Coat ½ in powdered cocoa and the other 1/2 confectioner's sugar.

Arrange in pairs on a tray and serve for your holiday party.

Remember to label them, as it is difficult to find balls that are vegan.

Sun Flower Power BonBon

This simple bonbon enables the busy individual to mix up a bonbon using one bowl or jar. Bonbon in a jar, is ideal for "on the go" snacks and between sporting events.

½ c	Sunflower seed butter
2 T	Honey
1 T	Coconut oil
1 T	Cocoa pwd
3 T	Astragalus

Mix the base ingredients, sunflower seed butter, honey and coconut oil together.

Add the cocoa into warm mixture. Then add Astragalus as a nutritive adaptogen for boosting immune system function.

You may store as bonbons mix in a sealed jar and eat directly out of it or Roll them in; sunflower seeds, coconut and/or cocoa powder.

Eat 2 T daily, especially during 3 o'clock slump for fuel and power.

Adding adaptogens into a nut butter base is one way to reduce the effects of stress and boost immune function. You may eat right from the container with a spoon as often as you'd like.

Testy Pumpkin Balls

In honor of men and testosterone this bonbon provides nourishment for the endocrine and reproductive systems.

1 c	Pumpkin seed butter
¼ c	Pumpkin seeds
¼ c	Lotus seeds, soaked in Amaretto until softened
1 T	Damiana pwd
3 T	Ashwagandha pwd
1 t	Cinnamon pwd
1 T	Maple syrup

Process first 3 ingredients in food processor
Add the powdered herbs
Drizzle the maple syrup into processor to get to right stiffness (consistency).
Roll mixture into large meatball size. Drop in two's onto waxed paper.

You may want to add more cinnamon or confectioner's sugar for rolling to get the preferred shade. Create different sizes and colors for diversity.

Tresie Cup

Reminiscent of a Reese's Cup, my Tresie Cup is a peanut butter and chocolate confection without fake sugars and hydrogenated fats. It is so nutritious you can call it food, not junk.

1 c	Coconut oil
1 c	Peanut Butter, creamy or crunchy
½ c	Honey
1 c	Cacao pwd
2 T	Cordyceps
2 T	Ashwagandha

Melt coconut oil over low heat in saucepan.
Add peanut butter, stir well to blend.
Take off heat and add honey. Stir
Add the Cacao powder with some nourishing adaptogen powders.
Mix well into warm nut blend.
Spoon into mini paper cupcake cups in mini muffin tin.
Refrigerate to set. Coconut oil will solidify when refrigerated
Keep them refrigerated as they melt quickly at room temperature.

Tresie Cups are a throwback to my childhood nickname "Tresie". Memories of the commercial jingles, "You got chocolate in my peanut butter, no you got your peanut better in my chocolate" stayed with me and influenced my favorite flavor combo. Enjoy the childhood pleasure blended into this recipe.

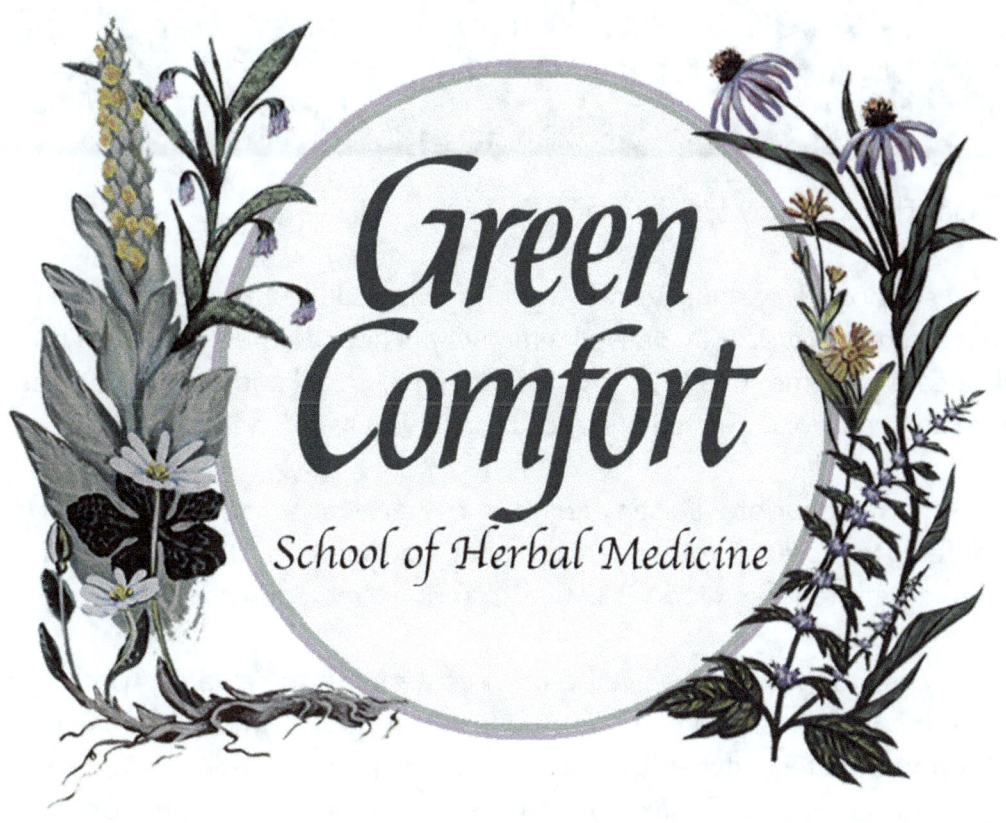

www.GreenComfortHerbSchool.com

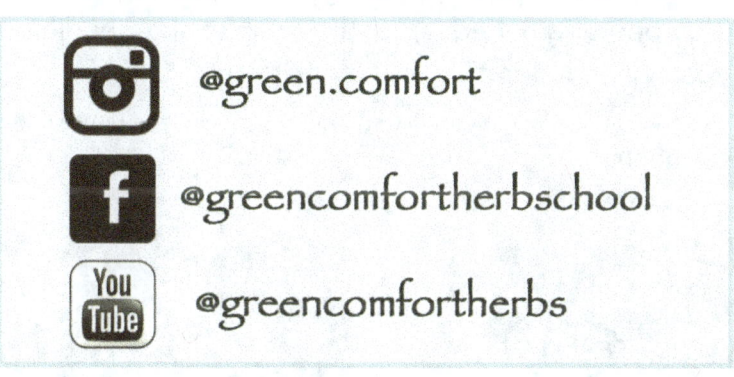

@green.comfort

@greencomfortherbschool

@greencomfortherbs

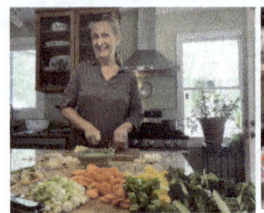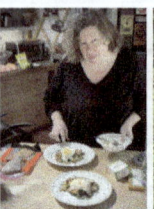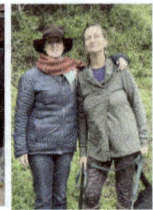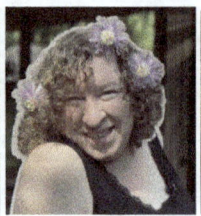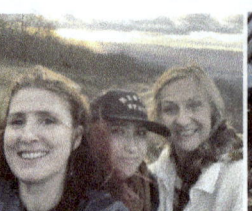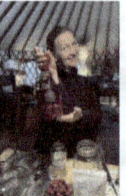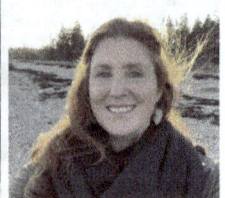

Special Thanks to my special crew!

To my supportive partner, Terry Waggener who edited this recipe book with great attention to detail. He wears many hats here at Green Comfort, he takes care of home, hearth, cooks for the herb school and even caretakes Mom so I can work. I am so blessed to have you as my dearest friend.

Thanks to my daughter Destiny for your love and inspiration. I love her desire to defend the forest, protect native plants, garden for sustainability and create a path to lessen food injustice. You bring me endless Joy!

For Tracie Little who drives five hours once a month to serve as Apothecary Apprentice. She insisted that I get the BonBon book to market and even helped run the test kitchen to try out some recipes. We appreciate the use of your photography. Thanks for your dedication and making me do it!

Big Thanks to Tara Griffin for the tireless work as graphic artist, project coordinator, book formatter and photographer. For all the hours going back and forth, incorporating my edits, for the push to the deadline. I am grateful for our 25 years of collaboration and friendship.

I love you so much,
♡Teresa

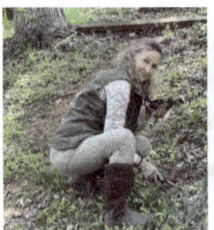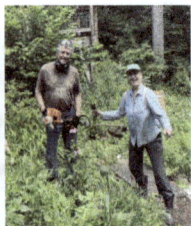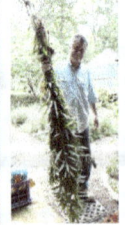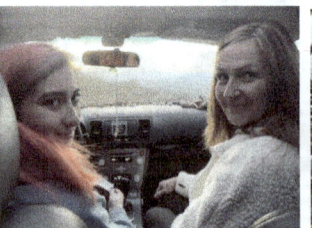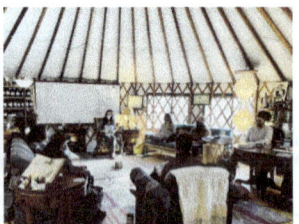

This book is full of
original herbal superfood
confections that will
sweeten your palate and
expand your heart